Understanding Periodontitis: A comprehensive guide to

Periodontal Disease for dentists, dental hygienists and dental patients.

(Revised Edition with current periodontal classification and review of 2017 World Workshop consensus on

Periodontal and Peri-implant diseases)

DR. NKEM OBIECHINA

AuthorHouse™
1663 Liberty Drive
Bloomington, IN 47403
www.authorhouse.com
Phone: 1 (800) 839-8640

Published by AuthorHouse 11/13/2018

ISBN: 978-1-4634-4611-6 (sc)

Library of Congress Control Number: 2011913624

Print information available on the last page.

Any people depicted in stock imagery provided by Thinkstock are models,
and such images are being used for illustrative purposes only.
Certain stock imagery © Thinkstock.

This book is printed on acid-free paper.

authorHOUSE®

TABLE OF CONTENTS:

Introduction

Periodontal disease is a chronic infection that affects bone and supporting tissue around teeth. If left untreated, periodontal disease can lead to tooth loss. The goal of this revised edition is to present information on the latest 2017 classification of periodontal and peri-implant disease and conditions, and contrast it to the existing 1999 classification in order to provide detailed information about understanding, diagnosing, making a prognosis about periodontal conditions and treating periodontal and peri-implant diseases.

This book looks at periodontal disease, and more specifically, the types and causes of plaque induced periodontitis. It also reviews factors including plaque and non-plaque related modulators that increase the risk of periodontal disease and how periodontal disease affects a person's periodontal, dental, and systemic health.

The goal is to provide a review for dentists, and hygienists about the current developments in diagnosis and treating periodontal disease, as well as to provide a detailed background about periodontitis for other people that want a better understanding about the causes and treatment of periodontitis.

Based on the NHANES III study of a representative sample to estimate periodontitis in 105.8 million civilian Americans between 1988 and 1994, fifty three percent of adults aged between thirty to ninety years had 3mm or more of attachment loss in at least one site, while about sixty four percent had probing depth in one site equal to or more than 3mm. Thirty five million adults thirty years and older based on the sample had periodontitis.[1]

The implications of not treating periodontitis go beyond detrimentally affecting dental health and tooth loss, and can severely affect systemic health as well. Strong correlations have been found between periodontal disease and systemic diseases such as coronary heart disease and diabetes.[7,15]

Severe periodontal disease is also correlated with worsening of diabetes and coronary heart disease. It also has implications for respiratory disease and can be correlated with low birth weight and pre-term birth in babies.[7] Periodontal disease not only presents a risk for the health of teeth, but also adversely affects systemic health.

Chapter 1: Periodontal Disease Overview

Periodontal disease is a condition that affects supporting tissue around the roots of teeth. Plaque induced periodontal disease is caused by bacterial plaque film which calcifies around teeth becoming tartar or calculus. Bacterial plaque can secrete an enzyme, collagenase, which can cause destruction of gingival tissue and bone.

As bacterial plaque accumulates in the mouth, inflammation results as the body releases cells such as neutrophils, monocytes and macrophages that target bacteria and attempt to engulf bacterial pathogens. The body also responds by releasing antibodies and T-cells to attack the bacterial pathogens. As inflammation progresses, the body also releases chemical mediators in response to the bacterial invasion such as cytokines like interleukin 1-Beta and prostaglandins to target bacterial plaque and to fight periodontal infection.

Excessive production of these mediators can become destructive, and instead can cause further break down of bone and connective tissue attachment. In essence, the protective process the body uses to fight infection goes awry, destroying bone and connective tissue.[19]

When inflammation occurring in a person's gums is at or bellow the gingival margin, but does not extend to the mucogingival junction or result in bone or attachment loss, this condition is called plaque induced gingivitis.[19] Plaque induced gingivitis is the initial manifestation of periodontal disease, but it does not always progress to become periodontitis and when reversed can result in periodontal health. It typically can present as bleeding during brushing and flossing or spontaneous bleeding in a person's gums.

Based on the characterization by the 2017 World workshop evaluating periodontal health, gingival diseases and conditions, three categories were recognized which included:[20]

1) Periodontal health which can occur on a healthy intact periodontium or on a reduced periodontium for stable periodontitis patients that have responded to therapy. Periodontal health can also occur in non periodontitis patients with reduced periodontium such as patients with recession.[20] Having health in a reduced periodontium is similar to an intact periodontium except that the patients with a reduced epithelium might have a higher chance of developing periodontitis compared to patients who have an intact periodontium due to their pre-existing attachment loss.[19]

2) Gingivitis related to dental biofilm. This category includes gingivitis affected by dental film alone, gingivitis mediated by local and systemic risk factors such as sex hormones, hyperglycemia, leukemia, smoking and malnutrition.[19]

Local factors affecting periodontal disease can include overhanging or subgingival restorations and hyposalivation that can result in plaque accumulation.[19]

3) Gingivitis can also be affected by drug induced gingival enlargements which affect the size of gingival tissue. The drugs that are primarily involved in causing tissue enlargement include antiepileptic drugs such as phenytoin, calcium channel blockers such as Nifedipine, Verapamil and Amlodipine, and immunoregulatory drugs such as cyclosporin and high dose oral contraceptives.[19]

In evaluating gingivitis, the variation of the 2017 classification from the 1999 classification deals with four components: 1) Describing the extent and severity of gingival inflammation, 2) Describing the extent and severity of gingival enlargement, 3) Reduction on taxonomy for gingivitis and 4) Discussing whether mild localized gingivitis should be considered a disease or variant of health.[19]

In response to characterizing severity and extent, the same definition for periodontitis was utilized where localized gingivitis involves less than 30% sites with gingival inflammation and generalized gingivitis involves from 30% or more sites in the mouth.[19]

The term "incipient gingivitis" was also coined, and is used to refer to gingivitis involving just a few sites with mild gingival inflammation, expressed by mild redness and delayed instead of spontaneous bleeding. While it is considered to be within the spectrum of "clinical health", it can result in localized gingivitis if it is not treated.[19]

In evaluating gingival enlargement, the extent of it is defined as localized or generalized based on the number of sites that are involved. While localized enlargement involves enlargement around a single tooth or group of teeth, generalized gingival enlargement affects the whole mouth.[19]

In defining severity of gingival enlargement, mild enlargement involves enlargement of the gingival papilla, moderate gingival enlargement involves enlargement of the gingival papilla and marginal gingiva while severe enlargement involves enlargement of the gingival papilla, gingival margin around teeth and attached gingiva.[19]

Once gingivitis is treated, usually by generalized cleaning or scaling, and oral hygiene measures such as brushing and flossing are back in place, it can be reversed. If left untreated, gingivitis can lead to loss of bone and supporting tissue attachment around teeth, known as periodontitis.

Symptoms of gingivitis can include: redness of gums, swelling, and bleeding in gums that is often spontaneous or that can occur during brushing and flossing. Gingivitis can also result in bad breath and gingival enlargement in gums. Sensitivity as a result of the inflammation can also be present in patients with plaque induced gingivitis.

Following initial phase of periodontal therapy including full mouth debridement or scaling and other therapy in addition to instituting good oral hygiene practices, gingivitis progression is often reversed. The remainder of this book as a result focuses on plaque induced periodontitis and non plaque related conditions that affect the periodontium as well as peri-implant diseases.

Currently, different forms of periodontitis exist. Based on the 1999 International workshop on periodontal diseases and conditions, seven categories of plaque induced periodontitis are widely recognized. An eight category involving developmental and acquired conditions was also described at the workshop. [2,3] The 1999 classification for plaque induced periodontitis included: chronic periodontitis, aggressive periodontitis, periodontitis associated with systemic disease, necrotizing periodontal diseases consisting of necrotizing ulcerative gingivitis (NUG) and necrotizing ulcerative periodontitis(NUP), periodontal disease related to abscesses, as well as periodontal disease associated with endodontic lesions. [2,3]

In 2017 the American Academy of Periodontology(AAP) and the European Federation of Periodontology(EFP) revised the classification for periodontitis to include Necrotizing Periodontal diseases, Periodontitis, and Periodontitis as a manifestation of systemic conditions. In addition, they created an additional classification involving other conditions that affect the periodontium.[20]

Necrotizing Periodontitis involves the subclassifications of:

1) Necrotizing Gingivitis: These involve acute infections of the gingiva characterized by gingival necrosis, bleeding and pain. NUG involves periodontal interdental necrosis, "punched out ulcerated papilla" and usually involves papillary and marginal gingiva.[21,22]

2) Necrotizing Periodontitis: This is an inflammatory condition of the periodontium that can be characterized by necrosis and ulcers of interdental papilla, gingival bleeding, halitosis, pain and rapid bone loss. It is usually associated with immunosuppression and can be present with pseudo membrane formation, lymphadenopathy and fever.[22]

3) Necrotizing Stomatitis: Severe inflammatory conditions in the gums and the oral cavity causing soft tissue necrosis that extends beyond the gingiva and bone denudation that can occur through the alveolar mucosa with areas of osteitis and formation of sequestration. It usually occurs in severely immunocompromised patients.[22]

The Periodontitis classification includes a combination of both localized and generalized Chronic and Aggressive periodontitis which were defined in the 1999 classification and will be reviewed separately later in the book. Periodontitis is categorized based on its severity, extent and risk of progression. Two new concepts were utilized to define it including the terms "Staging" and "Grading".[20]

1) Staging: This is based on the severity and complexity of managing periodontitis. It is determined by considering a number of variables including clinical attachment loss, probing depth, presence or absence of angular defects, furcation involvement, mobility and potential for tooth loss due to periodontitis. It involves four categories:[20]

Stage 1: Initial Periodontitis. It involves clinical attachment loss of 1-2mm, bone loss of only coronal third of root, and probing depth of 1-4mm. There is no tooth loss due to periodontal disease.[22]

Stage 2: Moderate Periodontitis. It involves clinical attachment loss of 3-4mm, bone loss in coronal third of root, probing depth of 1-5mm, mostly horizontal bone loss and no tooth loss due to periodontal disease.[22]

Stage 3: Severe periodontitis with potential for additional tooth loss. It involves clinical attachment loss of 5mm or more, bone loss extending to middle or apical third of root, probing depth of 6mm or more, class II or Class III furcation involvement and vertical bone loss. It involves loss of four or fewer teeth from periodontitis.[22]

Stage 4: Severe periodontitis with potential for loss of dentition. Involves clinical attachment loss of more than 5mm or more, bone loss extending to middle or apical third of root, probing depth of 6mm or more, class II or class III furcation involvement and vertical bone loss in addition to loss of five or more teeth from periodontal disease. There is a need for complex rehabilitation because these patients tend to have less than 20 teeth in both arches, and can present with bite collapse, and masticatory dysfunction.[22]

2) Grading involves additional information about biological characteristics of the periodontal condition, analysis of the risk of disease progression, rate of disease progression, anticipated outcomes of the treatment, and the assessment of the risk that the disease or its treatment would have on general health of the patient. It incorporates health status, environmental exposure such as smoking and level of metabolic control of diabetics and other patient dependent factors in assessing risk of periodontitis progression.[20] Grading involves three categories:

Grade A: Low risk of disease progression. It involves patients with no attachment loss for the past 5 years, less than .25% of bone loss per year, low level of disease progression with high bacterial biofilm and no risk factors such as smoking or diabetes present.[22]

Grade B: Involves moderate risk of progression. Patients have less than 2mm of attachment loss over 5 years and .25 to 1% of bone loss per year and periodontal destruction that is consistent with the biofilm that is present. The risk factors include smokers with less than 10 cigarettes per day and diabetics with glycosylated Hemoglobin A1c that is less than 7%.[22]

Grade C: Involves rapid risk of disease progression.[20] Patient have more than 2mm of attachment loss over 5 years, greater than 1% of bone loss per year, and destruction that is higher than the level of bacterial biofilm that is present in the mouth. Typically, there is rapid progression patterns of disease as well as molar and incisor involvement consistent with early onset periodontitis.[22] Risk factors are also present and include smokers of more that 10 cigarettes daily, as well as diabetics with glycosylated hemoglobin levels that are 7% or more.

3) Extent and distribution of periodontitis. When categorizing extent of periodontitis it can be classified as localized when less than 30% of sites are involved, while for sites with generalized periodontitis, 30% or more of the sites are involved. The pattern of the disease can involve incisor and molar distribution or show a general distribution to other teeth

in the mouth.[20,22]

A third classification of periodontitis includes periodontitis as a manifestation of systemic diseases. This category addresses systemic conditions that can manifest in the mouth and affect the periodontium. This classification did not change significantly from the 1999 classification reviewed later in the book and involves conditions such as Papillon Lefevre Syndrome, cyclic neutropenia and a number of other systemic disorders as well as some types of neoplasia. The only change made to this section is that diabetes was regrouped as a periodontal disease modulator rather than as periodontitis as a manifestation of systemic disease.[20]

Changes were made to the 1999 classification on Periodontal developmental and acquired deformities and conditions. It was combined with the categories on periodontal abscesses and endodontic lesions and reclassified in the 2017 report as Periodontal manifestations of systemic disease, developmental and acquired conditions. The category was divided into five additional subdivisions involving:

1) Systemic diseases and conditions affecting periodontal supporting tissues. A number of systemic diseases and condition affect periodontal tissue and can be categorized to include genetic disorders that affect host response and connective tissue, metabolic disorders, endocrine disorders such as diabetes mellitus, and inflammatory conditions.[23] They are not modified significantly from the 1999 classification so they will be reviewed in detailed later in the book. The only major change made is that both diabetes and smoking are classified as periodontal disease modifiers, and the extent of glycemic control and number of cigarettes smoked affects the grade of periodontal disease.[23]

2) Other periodontal conditions. Periodontal abscesses and Endodontic-Periodontal lesions were reclassified under this category in the 2017 workshop. Periodontal abscesses involve localized accumulation of pus within the gingival wall of the periodontal pocket.[22]The signs and symptoms associated with them include ovoid elevation in the gingiva along the lateral part of the root, bleeding on probing, pain, suppuration on probing, deep probing depth and tooth mobility.[22] Types of periodontal abscesses as well as their treatment is reviewed later in the book.

Endodontic-Periodontal lesions involve pathologic communication between the dental pulp and periodontal tissues that can be caused by caries, traumatic lesions that affect the pulp or by periodontal destruction that secondarily affects the root canal.[22] Signs include deep probing depth to the apex of teeth, or negative response to pulp tests, radiographic evidence of bone loss in the apical or furcation area, spontaneous pain, pain on palpation or percussion, suppuration, tooth mobility, and sinus tracts.[22] Root perforation, root fracture or external root resorption might also be present and can adversely impact the prognosis of the affected teeth.[22]

3) Mucogingival deformities and conditions occur around teeth and affect the periodontal apparatus.[23]

- Gingival phenotype refers to a term that combines both thickness of tissue around teeth in three dimensions (soft tissue phenotype) and thickness of bone buccal plate (bone morphotype). It was initially called Biotype, but the 2017 classification made a recommendation for the change to the term "gingival phenotype". It is measured directly using a periodontal probe inserted in the sulcus with 1mm or less thickness and probe visibility indicating a thin phenotype, and more that 1mm thickness with no probe visible for a thick gingival phenotype.[23]

- Gingival or soft tissue recession involves an apical shift of gingival margin that is caused by factors such as subgingival restorations in sites with thin phenotypes or pathology. Patients that are receiving orthodontic therapy can have recession especially if teeth are being proclined.[23]

- Lack of gingiva. Lack of keratinized gingival tissue does not always signal potential inflammation or periodontal damage especially for patients with good oral hygiene.

- Decreased vestibular depth can cause mucogingival problems with teeth that are associated with the site without necessarily causing recession.[23]

- Ectopic frenum attachment or position can cause gingival recession over time especially for teeth with thin gingival phenotype.[23]

- Gingival excess/overgrowth can result from medications such as calcium channel blockers, anti-transplant rejection drugs and antiepileptic drugs as well as from inflammation from local factors such as sub-gingival restorations, altered passive eruption, and pathology. They will be reviewed in detail in the chapter dealing with developmental and acquired conditions.

- Condition of the exposed root surface is usually noted in assessing roots with recession or mucogingival problems. The goal is to observe for the presence of caries, and other pathologic conditions as well as anatomic conditions that could alter the surface of the root making it more prone to periodontal damage such as cemental tears, and enamel projections, or the presence of fenestration or dehiscence defects.

- Abnormal gingival color can occur due to hypersensitivity to dental materials which can appear as localized inflammation or discoloration in the gums.[23]

4) Traumatic occlusal forces: A consensus was made by the 2017 World Workshop to rename excessive occlusal force as Traumatic occlusal forces, and use it to characterize any force that causes damage to the periodontal apparatus.[23] Indications of traumatic occlusal forces can include: fremitus, tooth mobility, tooth sensitivity, excessive occlusal wear, tooth migration, pain on mastication, teeth fracture, widened periodontal ligament space (PDL), root resorption and hyper-cementosis.[23,24] The workshop also redefined occlusal trauma as the response to injury caused to the periodontal apparatus.

a) Primary occlusal trauma: Injury resulting in tissue changes within the attachment apparatus including PDL, alveolar bone, and cementum around a tooth or teeth with intact periodontium. The teeth have normal bone and clinical attachment level with excessive forces present.[24]

b) Secondary occlusal trauma: This involves tissue changes in response to injury from normal or excessive force applied to teeth with reduced periodontium. It occurs in the presence of attachment loss, bone loss and normal or excessive occlusal forces.[24]

c) Orthodontic forces: A number of studies have shown that teeth with reduced but healthy periodontal support in the presence of good oral hygiene practices can be able to have successful orthodontic therapy without compromising the periodontal support around the teeth.[23] In some instances, orthodontic forces can be able to cause damage in the form of root resorption, gingival recession and alveolar bone loss.[23]

5) Prosthesis and tooth related factors that modify or predispose to plaque-induced gingival disease are divided into two categories:[20]

-Localized tooth related factors: These include conditions that change root anatomy such as cervical projections, root fractures, cervical root resorption, cemental tears, root proximity and altered passive eruption involving coronal location of the gingival margin. [20]These conditions can cause localized loss of attachment or bone, or pseudo pocketing in the area.

-Localized dental prosthesis related factors: These conditions deal with damage to the periodontium as a result of restorations or restorative materials.[23] They can occur when restorations are placed sub-gingivally affecting the supra-crestal attached tissues(renamed by the 2017 periodontal disease workshop, formerly known as biologic width).[23] They can also cause localized inflammation due to indirect restorations or reactions and hypersensitivity to restorative materials.[23]

Chapter 2: Diagnosing Periodontal disease

Typically, the most common sign that is found with periodontal disease is bleeding that can be spontaneous or occur during brushing and flossing. Other indications of the presence of periodontal disease can also include changes in the form of gum tissue such as recession or gingival enlargement, swelling in gums, as well as spacing or crowding in teeth. Symptoms such as food impaction in between teeth following meals, tooth mobility, sensitivity or dull throbbing pain around a person's gums may also be indications of underlying periodontal disease. Any of these signs and symptoms being present may indicate a need for periodontal examination and periodontal treatment.

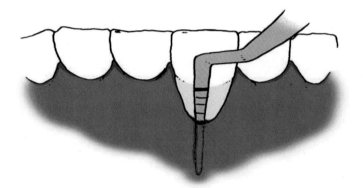

Fig. 1: Signs of periodontal disease include bleeding, redness in gums, recession and gingival swelling.

Diagnosis of periodontal disease involves a periodontal exam which measures both the depth of periodontal pockets around teeth, and the actual loss of tissue attachment that is missing from the tooth. Probing depth refers to a measurement from the gingival margin to the base of the gingival crevice using a periodontal probe. Clinical attachment loss measures from a fixed point on a tooth such as the cemento-enamel junction to the base of the gingival crevice. These measurements are compared against clinical findings from a clinical exam as well as the findings that are present on a full series of x-rays in order to give an accurate diagnosis of a person's periodontal condition.

Periodontal disease was also classified based on recommendations made by American Dental Association (ADA) and Academy of Periodontology (AAP). This previous classification is based on the severity of periodontal disease using both probing depth measurements, clinical attachment level and dental x-rays. These guidelines were made to demarcate various case types of periodontal disease and are also utilized by dental insurance companies in classifying periodontal disease progression.

Based on their classification, **Case type 1** refers to Gingivitis. When a person has gingivitis, clinically, there may be bleeding on probing. Gums may also appear red and inflamed, but no connective tissue attachment loss or bone loss occurs as a result of gingivitis. Following appropriate therapy and institution of oral hygiene, gingivitis can be resolved.

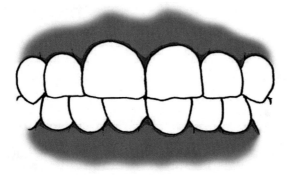

Fig. 2 and Fig. 3: Gingivitis showing inflammation and redness in gums

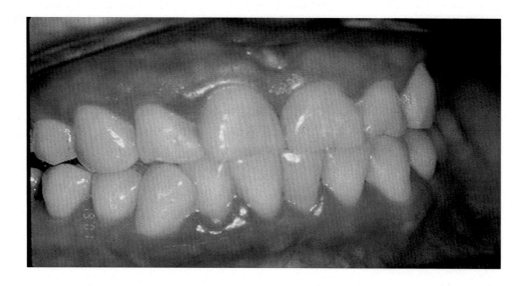

Case Type II refers to mild periodontitis. It manifests as bleeding on probing, in addition to probing depth of 3-4mm. There might also be recession, and mild furcation involvement as well due to mild periodontitis. Findings on x-rays can be able to identify horizontal bone loss, and bone level typically within 3-4mm from the cemento-enamel junction.

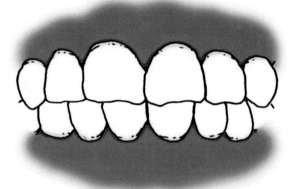

Fig.4: Early Periodontitis showing inflammation, recession and plaque

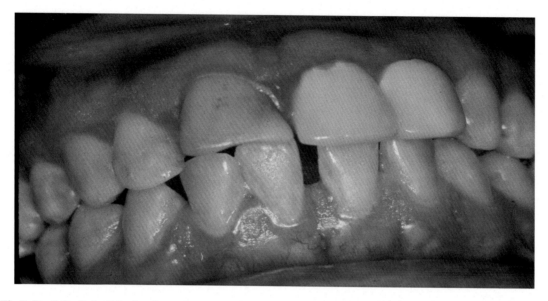

Fig.5: Early Periodontitis showing redness and edematous consistency of gingival tissues due to inflammation

Case type III is classified as moderate periodontitis. Teeth that are affected have probing depth of 4-6mm, bleeding during probing measurements, furcation involvement and tooth mobility. Radiographic findings often include bone loss that is 4-6mm from the CEJ around the roots of teeth. Moderate to severe amount bone loss is typically present resulting in a crown to root ratio that can approach 1:1, with root size being equal to the amount of tooth structure that is present in the mouth. Therefore, there is diminished support and stability around teeth.

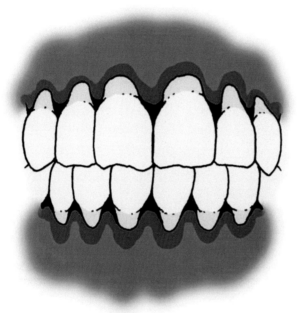

Fig.6: Moderate periodontitis showing recession, attachment loss, and inflammation

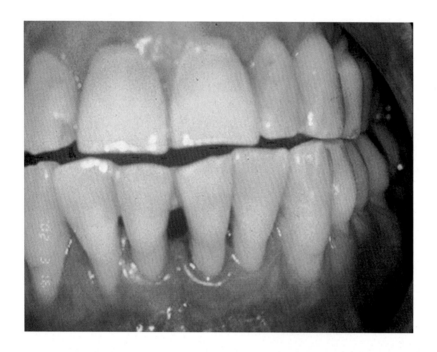

Fig.7: Moderate periodontitis showing recession and inflammation

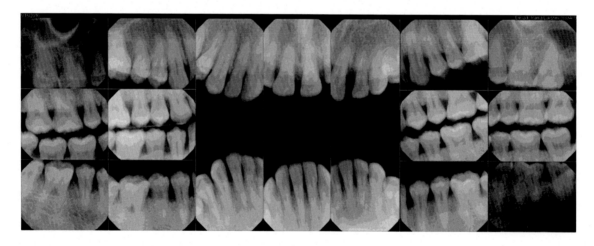

Fig.8: X-rays showing bone loss associated with moderate periodontitis

Case Type IV is referred to as advanced periodontitis. Probing depth is typically more that 6mm, with some teeth that can have furcation involvement that can extend from one side of the tooth to the opposite side (grade III furcation involvement), and mobility that is severe in nature. On dental x-rays, there is horizontal as well as vertical bone loss. Bone loss around teeth with advanced periodontitis is usually greater than 6mm.

The crown to root ratio can approach 2:1, meaning that often twice as much tooth structure is present in the mouth compared to the root underneath. When advanced periodontitis occurs, this means that the support around a tooth has been severely compromised, and the stability and prognosis of the tooth have become diminished as a result of it.

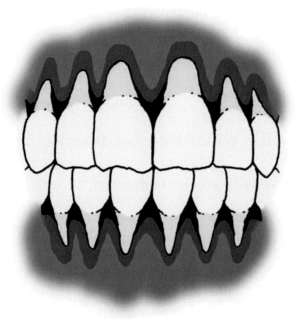

Fig.9: Clinical findings associated with advanced Periodontitis

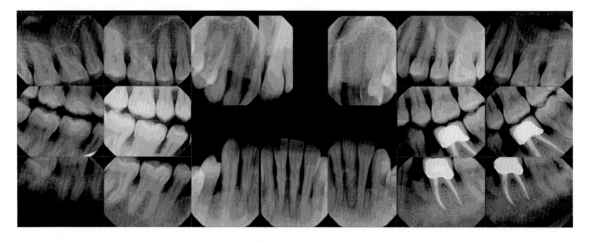

Fig.10: X-rays showing severe bone loss associated with advanced Periodontitis

Based on the 1999 classification system of periodontal disease, dental plaque induced gingival diseases can include gingivitis, endocrine related disease such as pregnancy gingivitis, and diabetes mellitus, drug induced gingival diseases such as medication induced gingival overgrowth and gingival diseases that are related to nutritional deficiencies. [3]

Non plaque induced gingival conditions can include gingival manifestations from non-periodontal pathogens such as viruses and the viral organism causing herpetic gingiva-stomatitis, fungal infections such as candidiasis as well as streptococcal infections. Systemic conditions such as Pemphigus and Lupus erythematous can also have oral implications and manifest as non-plaque induced lesions. Allergies to food, toothpastes and mouthwashes, as well as trauma from physical, chemical or thermal injury can result in gingival lesions, and are classified as non-plaque induced gingival conditions because though they are not linked to plaque induced periodontal diseases, they are able to manifest as periodontal lesions in the mouth.[3]

In 2017, gingival plaque induced conditions were revised to include: 1) Periodontal health and gingival health on intact or reduced epithelium, 2) Gingivitis that is biofilm induced including conditions caused by biofilm only, and 3) those associated with biofilm as well as with systemic risk factors such as conditions caused by sex steroid hormones, hyperglycemia, leukemia, smoking and malnutrition, and local factors such as overhanging or subgingival restorations, and hyposalivation as well as drug induced gingival overgrowth.

The 2017 World Workshop consensus modified gingival conditions that are not biofilm induced to include systemic diseases linked to genetic disorders, inflammatory or immune conditions, neoplasms, traumatic lesions and pigmentation. The taxonomy of gingival conditions was also revised to remove terms such as "oral contraceptive induced gingivitis", and "ascorbic acid induced gingivitis" as separate categories.[19]

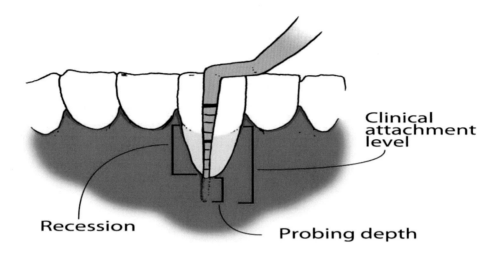

Fig.11: Parameters used to measure periodontal disease

Mild periodontal attachment destruction is believed to be present when there is 1-2mm of clinical attachment loss around a tooth. Moderate periodontal destruction occurs when 3-4mm of clinical attachment loss occurs around the roots of teeth. Severe periodontal destruction occurs when 5mm or more of attachment loss occurs around the root of a tooth. Both attachment loss measurements and probing depth measures can be used to classify the severity of periodontal destruction and is now categorized using the term "staging" as reviewed earlier with four stages existing for categorizing disease severity.[20]

Periodontal disease typically occurs with a pattern of some sites in the mouth breaking down while other sites in the mouth stay stable at a given time. As a result, it can be classified by its extent. When more than thirty percent of the sites in the mouth are affected, the extent of the periodontal disease is classified as generalized. Localized periodontitis refers to periodontal involvement of less than thirty percent of sites in the mouth.

In recommending periodontal therapy for a patient, identifying the type and stage of periodontal disease, and grade of periodontal disease all play an important role in adequately diagnosing and treating a patient's periodontal condition and preventing further progression of the disease.

Chapter 3: Chronic Periodontitis (Reclassified as Periodontitis)

The most prevalent form of periodontitis is chronic periodontitis. Two major forms of chronic periodontitis exist, which are generalized and localized chronic periodontitis. Patients who have chronic periodontitis typically have a significant amount of local causative factors that are causing periodontal disease such as plaque and tartar deposits. The level of plaque and tartar deposits matches the level of destruction in the periodontal tissues, and the amount of bone loss present on x-rays usually corresponds to the amount of periodontal disease present.

People with chronic periodontitis are usually adults who are thirty years and older who present with plaque and tartar deposits on their teeth. Factors such as smoking and systemic conditions like diabetes are able to affect and modulate the extent and grade of chronic periodontitis. Radiographic assessment tends to reveal horizontal bone loss rather than vertical patterns of bone loss, although vertical bone loss can occur with chronic periodontitis.

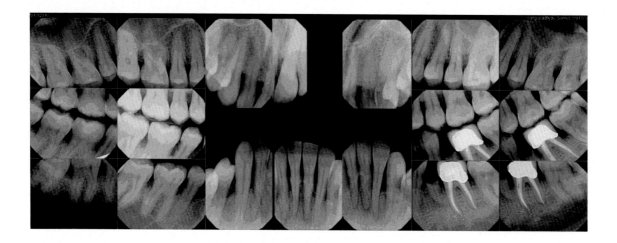

Fig.12: X-rays showing bone loss associated with chronic periodontitis

Bacterial analysis shows that while the major pathogens that cause periodontal disease are typically present, they are variable in nature. The typical bacteria that are responsible for causing chronic periodontitis are: P. gingivalis, E.corredens, B. forsythus, C. rectus, E. nodatum, P. micros, P.intermedia, S.intermedia and Treponema species.[12] These bacterial pathogens are found in varying amounts in people with chronic periodontitis.

In addition, there is not really any major genetic aggregation for chronic periodontitis, which means that members of the same family do not typically manifest traits for chronic periodontitis unlike the familial pattern that is found in aggressive periodontitis.

Probing depth formation and loss of clinical attachment is typically slower in nature compared to aggressive periodontitis, which means that loss of bone on x-rays and probing depth formation, as well as progression of probing depth measures occur over a longer period of time. Pocket depth occurring as a result of periodontitis represents an inflammatory response that causes swelling of gingival tissue at the top of the pocket, and also loss of collagen attachment to the tooth at the base of the pocket.[11] Deeper pockets tend to impede access for plaque removal, and measurements at the base of a periodontal pocket can remain constant, or increase over time. [11]

With regard to the extent of chronic periodontitis, both types of chronic periodontitis have the same manifestations, with the only varying feature being the extent of the two diseases. Localized chronic periodontitis refers to periodontitis that affects less than thirty percent of the sites, while generalized chronic periodontitis affects thirty or more percent of sites on teeth in the mouth.

Periodontal therapy to treat chronic periodontitis typically involves initial therapy comprised of scaling and root planning and sometimes locally delivered chemotherapeutic agents such as Arrestin and Chlorhexidine. The main goal of initial therapy is to reduce inflammation and help to reduce probing depth in order to prevent further progression of periodontal disease.

When moderate or advanced chronic periodontitis is diagnosed, involving probing depth of 5mm and more, there is a need for surgical intervention to reduce probing depth around teeth as well as to get access for further removal of bacterial plaque. Flap surgery and osseous surgery are typically performed to remove bacterial plaque and for probing depth reduction. Guided tissue regeneration surgery utilizing

bone grafts and membranes may also be necessary in order to regain lost

periodontal support around teeth.

Chapter 4: Aggressive Periodontitis (Reclassified as Periodontitis)

Aggressive periodontitis is another major form of periodontitis, which is less prevalent than chronic periodontitis and affects a younger population of people who are typically under the age of thirty. The pattern of bone and attachment loss around teeth is very rapid, and a significant amount of bone and attachment can be lost in a very short period of time.

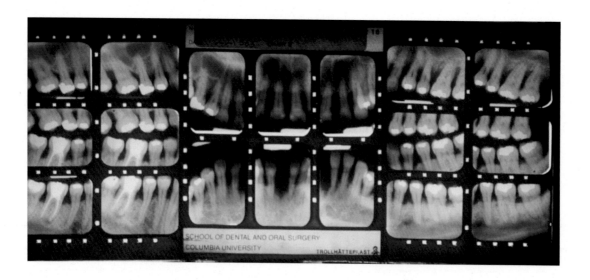

Fig.13: X-rays showing bone loss associated with Aggressive generalized periodontitis

Typically, the level of clinical attachment loss and probing depth levels does not coincide with the amount of plaque and calculus that is present. People with aggressive periodontitis have very little plaque and calculus deposits present in comparison to the extent of their periodontal destruction, but at the same time have rapidly occurring bone and attachment loss around their teeth.

A combination of the lack of plaque and tartar and the aggressive nature of destruction can often leave the patient unaware of the condition until severe periodontal destruction has occurred. People with aggressive periodontitis are usually systemically healthy, and do not have systemic conditions such as diabetes and heart disease that can contribute to the manifestation of periodontal disease. The typical person with this condition is a young adult who has no contributing factors and very little plaque or tartar deposits present, but at the same time manifests with a significant amount of periodontal destruction present.

People with Aggressive periodontitis often have malfunction of monocytes, macrophages and neutrophils, with excessive amounts of inflammatory phenotypes being present on these cells. As a result, there is an excessive accumulation of inflammatory bi- products that can cause further bone loss and loss of attachment. [2]

There is also an impairment in how neutrophils can be able to engulf and destroy invading bacterial cells, with decreased ability of neutrophils to be able to do this. There are also increased levels of PGE2 and IL-1B in gingival-crevicular fluid (GCF) and serum of people with aggressive periodontitis, these two mediators are usually associated with inflammation and periodontal break down.[2]

Two major bacteria are typically found in most people with aggressive periodontitis. These bacteria include Actinobacillus actinomycemcomitans (Aa) and Porphomonas gingivalis (Pg). Both bacteria are responsible for the severe destruction that occurs during aggressive periodontitis.[12]

Unlike in chronic periodontitis where the bacteria pattern varies, either bacteria or both are typically present in the gums of people with aggressive periodontitis. Periodontal destruction is very quick and happens within a very short time. Looking on radiographs would reveal vertical patterns of bone loss that can be severe in nature.

Two types of aggressive periodontitis exist: generalized and localized aggressive periodontitis. Both types have varying characteristics and manifest as different diseases.

Localized aggressive periodontitis typically affects only first molars and incisors. Its onset is in the earlier part of life, typically, pre pubertal to pubertal age, there is also a strong antibody response to bacterial invasion, and the IgG2 antibody is the antibody most often involved in the response.[2]

Generalized aggressive periodontitis affects people who are under the age of thirty years. There is a poor serum antibody response to bacterial invasion, and at least three other permanent teeth which are not first molars and incisors are involved. Periodontal destruction is episodic with random bursts of destructive activity followed by a period of quiescence.[2]

Treatment of Aggressive periodontitis requires focused periodontal therapy often involving surgery, multiple bone grafts and guided tissue regeneration, extraction of hopeless teeth, in combination with antibiotic therapy. Because the bacterial strains that cause this condition are very virulent, surgery in addition to antibiotics is needed in order to reduce their presence in gums.

Chapter 5: Periodontitis that is associated with systemic conditions.

Some systemic conditions can also be related to periodontitis. These include hematological disorders like acquired Neutropenia, and genetic disorders such as Papillon LeFevre sydrome, and Crohn's disease, leukocyte adhesion deficiency, agranulocytosis, lazy leukocyte syndrome, Hypogamma globunemia, Chediak -Higashi Syndrome, Glycogen storage diseases, infantile genetic agranulocytosis, and Ehler Danlos syndrome(collagen type II, type VIII, and type VII) [2] Diabetes was considered a condition that had periodontal manifestations based on the 1999 classification but was revised in the 2017 classification as a modulator of periodontitis, and glycemic control was utilized in combination with number of cigarettes smoke to characterize risk affecting the grade of periodontitis.[20]

Systemic diseases such as acquired Neutropenia which involves decreased neutrophil counts over more than a six month period can modify the body's defense mechanism, resulting in a reduced resistance against bacterial infections and can manifest periodontally as rapid loss of support around teeth and tooth loss.

Genetic conditions such as Papillon Lefevre syndrome, an autonomic recessive disorder caused by Cathepsin C deficiency that is characterized by palmo-planter hyperkeratosis and early onset periodontitis is one of the disorders that can also have oral implications. Early onset periodontitis and tooth loss might be the first indications of the presence of this disorder, it is therefore extremely important not to ignore these manifestations when they are present, and instead to complete the necessary screening for the condition.

Other genetic conditions such as leukocyte adhesion syndrome, Chediak Higashi syndrome, glycogen storage diseases, and infantile agranulocytosis, are disorders affecting neutrophil number and function, and can also result in early loss of teeth and susceptibility to bacterial infections. These as well as the other systemic conditions mentioned can present themselves as periodontitis, and often result in early periodontitis in younger patients, and premature tooth loss.

Ehler danlos syndrome, a systemic condition involving defects in connective tissue, results in hyper extensive skin as well as periodontal problems in affected individuals. Hypo-phosphatasia also manifests as periodontitis and is a condition caused by an excessive resorption of bone due to problems with bone mineralization caused by deficiency in alkaline phosphatase enzyme.

Because these systemic conditions can manifest orally in the mouth, performing routine blood tests and urine analysis to screen for the systemic condition present is a major step in accurately diagnosing and treating the underlying systemic condition.

Other systemic conditions like diabetes, result in an exaggerated response to the monocyte phenotype, and as a result, in the mouth, results in a more severe inflammatory response. As diabetic condition worsens typically, there is a corresponding break down in periodontal condition.[15] It was therefore reclassified as a modulator of periodontitis by the 2017 World workshop.[20]

Uncontrolled diabetics have a 2.9 fold chance of having severe periodontitis compared to controlled diabetics and healthy individuals. A number of recent studies have also shown that as periodontal condition improves the diabetic control of individuals improves and vice versa, when diabetic control improves, there is an improvement in periodontal health.[15]

These findings led to the recommendation made in 2009 by the International diabetes federation, and World dental federation calling for periodontal screening and treatment for diabetic patients and also routine screenings from periodontitis patients to rule out diabetes.

The improvement of diabetic control following institution of appropriate periodontal therapy also indicates the strength of the periodontal link to systemic health, and once again stresses how important it is not to ignore symptoms present in the mouth that could be manifestations of systemic disorders in other parts of the body.

Chapter 6: Periodontal Disease that is related to Periodontal abscesses (Reclassified as Other periodontal conditions that affect the periodontium)

Dental abscesses occur as a result of bacterial invasion around a tooth and its supporting structures. As the body mounts a response against the bacterial pathogens, and attempts to isolate it, an abscess results. Abscesses often contain pus, and can be isolated to a specific region of the mouth. Swelling from dental abscesses can be intra-oral or extra-oral depending on the origin of the abscess.

Dental abscesses can either be classified as periodontal, involving supporting tissues around teeth, or endodontic in origin, originating from the infection of the pulp of teeth.

Periodontal abscesses which result from bacterial invasion of periodontal tissue can manifest as periodontitis. Typically, the abscess is localized to the gums, but can sometimes involve bone and supporting connective tissue around a tooth.

When an abscess affects just the gums it is called a gingival abscess because it originates and remains in gum tissue and does not extend to the supporting tissue underneath.[13]

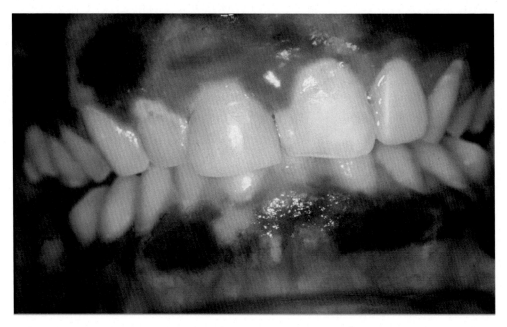

Fig. 14: Gingival Abscess

Periodontal abscesses occur when gingival abscesses extend from the gums into bone and connective tissue attachment underneath.[13] They are defined as acute lesions that involve accumulation of pus within the gingival wall of the periodontal pocket and rapid tissue destruction with potential risk of systemic dissemination.[22]

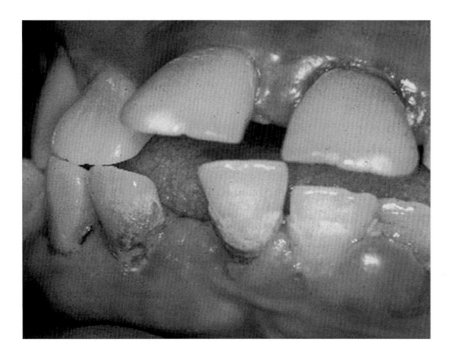

Fig.15: Periodontal abscess

Periodontal abscesses that are associated with partially erupted teeth, and result from inflammation of tissue around an erupting tooth are called peri-coronal abscesses. They result from an infection in teeth that have peri-coronitis. As a result of the gingival tissue around the teeth getting inflamed and irritated, it results in the formation of a fluctuant abscess.

Typically, peri-coronal abscesses most often occur in erupting third molars. Pain can start to occur when the abscess spreads into surrounding tissue around the tooth.

Treatment of periodontal abscesses involves gingival curettage, irrigation with chlorhexidine rinse, followed by systemic antibiotics. After gingival curettage, placement of a suture inter-proximally might be necessary to maintain the blood clot in the case of periodontal abscesses, in order to further enhance healing following removal of the tissue associated with the abscess.[13]

Once the abscess is resolved, institution of the appropriate periodontal therapy becomes necessary. For patients with peri-coronal abscess formation, the affected wisdom tooth should have to be removed as soon as the antibiotic therapy has been completed.

Chapter 7: Periodontitis related to Endodontic Abscesses (Reclassified under Other conditions affecting the Periodontium)

Endodontic abscesses occur when bacterial infection extends beyond the pulp and canals of a tooth into surrounding tissue. They are typically caused by dental caries that leads to an infected pulp, but can also occur as a result of mechanical injury to the pulp. Failure to treat the infection can lead to the abscess extending beyond the apex of a tooth and forming a cavity filled with pus. This cavity can be readily visualized with x-rays, and over time can be walled off by a fibrous sac called a granuloma.

Swelling resulting from endodontic abscesses can be both intra-oral, visible inside of the mouth, or extra oral, visible outside the face. Two types of endodontic abscesses can occur; acute abscesses that tend to occur shortly after bacterial invasion and cause severe pain, swelling and often fever, and chronic abscesses which are painless in nature and occur over a period of time, and over time can become granulomas or peri-apical cysts.

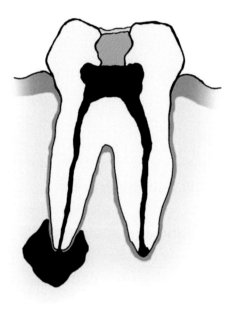

Fig.17: Endodontic Abscess

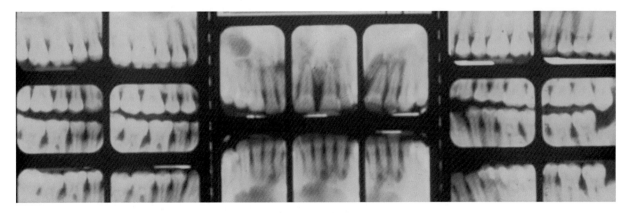

Fig.18: X-rays showing multiple peri-apical abscesses, granulomas and peri-apical cysts

Typically, acute abscesses that result from bacterial invasion of roots are extremely painful. Patients are often alerted to this condition as a result of the pain and swelling. The diagnosis is usually confirmed by an x-ray of the tooth and pulp tests, and usually manifests as a radiolucency bellow the root of a tooth.

Endodontic abscesses can cause damage to bone and underlying tissue supporting a tooth sometimes resulting in bone and attachment loss that is seen in periodontitis. Diagnosing and treating the cause of the abscess is therefore essential to maintaining the periodontal health of a tooth.

Treatment of endodontic abscesses usually involves antibiotic therapy, root-canal therapy or re-treatment of previous root canal performed after incision and drainage of the swelling when indicated. If the teeth also have periodontal involvement, completion of appropriate periodontal therapy is initiated following root canal therapy. For teeth with extensive bone loss or severe mobility present, the cause of action required would be to extract the tooth following antibiotic therapy.

Chapter 8: Acquired and Developmental conditions affecting periodontal health

A number of periodontal conditions can be able to affect periodontal health. These conditions can either be developmental or acquired. Developmental conditions are abnormalities in the form of gingival tissue that people are born with. These irregularities manifest in tooth structure and underlying gum tissue, although in some instances, they may not adversely affect gingival health, however in most instances, they result in the region of the mouth where they are located becoming more prone to periodontal break down.[10]

Ectopic frenal attachments are one of these conditions that can be able to adversely affect the health of teeth. Over time because the frenum is erroneously located higher on gingival attached tissue rather than mucosal tissue, attached tissue can be lost with time causing gingival recession around the tooth.

Multi-rooted teeth which have furcations where the roots separate can also be more prone to periodontal involvement than single rooted teeth for patients that do not have a molar/incisor disease distribution. This is because plaque accumulating around the furcation area can be difficult to remove, and can result in bone loss occurring in the furcation area as a result. Single rooted teeth are less likely to have periodontal involvement compared to multi rooted teeth because they lack furcations, and therefore have better access for oral hygiene performance.

Stillman's clefts are areas around teeth which occur developmentally that manifest as deficiencies in gum tissue around teeth, they occur usually when there is apical migration of gingival tissue. Typically, no treatment is required except in the cases where there is no attached gingival tissue around teeth, or when they are located in esthetic areas in the mouth.

Dehiscences are other anatomic factors that can be able to affect periodontal condition. Dehiscences are defects in bone that are not caused by bacterial plaque. The bone covering the root of a tooth might be thin and as a result, the root is exposed in the area. These root exposures occurring due to lack of bone covering the roots of teeth are called dehiscences. When treatment is indicated, the goal of therapy in the area is to attempt to regain the bone that was lost in the area using guided tissue regeneration.

Other gingival developmental conditions that affect location of the muco-gingival junction include altered passive eruption. Gingival tissue around teeth can erupt slower in some teeth than other teeth. As a result, the teeth appear to have an increased amount of gum tissue covering the tooth than should be present.

This can lead to probing depth around teeth without loss of attachment or bone (pseudo-pocketing) and in some instances there is excessive amount of gum tissue covering the crown of teeth "gummy smiles". Treatment when indicated is gingivectomy or gingivoplasty procedure.

In instances when there is also inadequate sulcus space and supra-crestal attached tissue (biologic width) could be violated, crown lengthening or osseous surgery can also be performed to increase the clinical length of teeth.

Non anatomic factors that can affect periodontal health can include local factors and host susceptibility factors that can increase risk of periodontal disease. The local factors include abrasion and cemental tears, recession, overhanging restorations, braces or orthodontic devices, malocclusion and restorative margins which impinge on the biological width, and over contoured restorations.[10]

Abrasion and cemental tears which modify the surface of the root can be able to increase bacterial accumulation and retention and as a result, more loss of clinical attachment results in such areas compared to smooth root surfaces.[10]

Overhanging and over contoured restorations can make oral hygiene access very difficult. In the case of overhanging restorations, the restorations can serve as plaque traps, allowing bacteria to accumulate underneath them causing bone and attachment loss in the area as a result. They should be replaced with adequate restorations when noted.

Orthodontics devices and braces can also limit access for oral hygiene, therefore a stricter oral hygiene regimen is recommended in order to remove plaque from braces and other orthodontic appliances.

Occlusal trauma can affect the periodontal attachment around teeth. Traumatic occlusal force was coined to define excessive force applied to the periodontal attachment apparatus.[23]Two forms of occlusal responses occur due to traumatic occlusion. Primary occlusal trauma occurs as a result of excessive occlusal force on teeth with healthy periodontal tissue, such as a tooth with a restoration with high occlusal contacts, or an individual that grinds their teeth at night.

Secondary occlusal trauma occurs a result of normal forces on weakened periodontal support, such as mastication forces on teeth with extensive bone loss. It can also occur due to excessive trauma to teeth that have reduced periodontal support due to attachment loss and bone

loss.[23] With regard to occlusal forces, the cause of the trauma should be

identified and addressed prior to surgical periodontal therapy.

Chapter 9: Host susceptibility factors affecting periodontal disease

Factors that affect and modulate periodontal health can include smoking, osteoporosis or osteopenia, diabetes, heart disease, and hormonal changes such as use of high potency oral contraceptives, pregnancy and menopause.

A number of factors affect host susceptibility to periodontal disease such as smoking, which is the number one modulator of periodontal disease. Smoking has been found to adversely affect both the risk and the severity of periodontal disease. Smokers also have been found to lose more teeth than non-smokers, about forty two percent of smokers compared to twenty percent of non-smokers had lost all their teeth by the age of 65 years. Smokers were also found to be four times more likely than non-smokers to have periodontitis.[16]

Prior smokers also were more at risk of having periodontitis than non- smokers with the risk decreasing as the number of years since smoking increased. [16]

Other factors such as osteoporosis have also been found to be able to increase risk of periodontitis. Women with osteoporosis were also found to have increased amount of bone loss as well as tooth loss due to the decreased density in their bones. A study on 1265 post- menopausal women found that those with periodontal bacterial pathogens in their mouth were more likely to have bone loss and tooth loss than those without periodontal plaque in their mouth.[5]

Hormonal changes can also have an effect on periodontal disease risk. Studies on young women taking oral contraceptives, found that young women taking certain high estrogen based oral contraceptives were more likely to have an increase in gingival bleeding compared to other women that were not taking contraceptives.[14] Hence, certain types of high concentration birth control pills make women more prone to periodontal inflammation and periodontal disease.

Studies conducted to evaluate impact of estrogen deficiency and hormone replacement in menopausal women found that estrogen replacement is associated with decreased gingival inflammation and clinical attachment loss for women with osteoporosis in early menopause, hence the conclusion that hormone replacement therapy can help reduce risk of periodontal disease for women in menopause. [14]

Other conditions such as diabetes mellitus and cardiovascular disease have been found to have links with periodontal disease. Treatment of periodontal disease has been shown to improve the level of high blood pressure and diabetic control for periodontitis patients. As a result recommendations were made for screening of periodontitis in this population of patients. [7, 15]

Chapter 10: Necrotising Periodontal Diseases

Necrotizing Periodontal Diseases are made up of necrotizing ulcerative gingivitis (NUG) and necrotizing ulcerative periodontitis (NUP) and Necrotizing stomatitis.[22] Necrotizing ulcerative gingivitis (NUG) is an acute infection of the gums that does not involve other periodontal tissues. It is characterized by necrosis of the gums, ulceration and blunting of the inter-proximal papilla, and also bright red gums which bleed on light probing, in addition to halitosis.

Factors such as smoking, stress, malnutrition especially in children and poor oral hygiene can exacerbate necrotizing ulcerative gingivitis (NUG). It is also a symptom that occurs frequently in immuno-suppressed individuals.

Treatment for NUG involves irrigation utilizing chlorhexidine mouth rinse and other oral rinses, debridement of the necrotic tissue, institution of oral hygiene measures, as well as pain medications in cases where patients have discomfort.

Necrotizing ulcerative periodontitis (NUP) is characterized by very aggressive bone and attachment loss. It is a very rapidly progressing condition that is typically associated with extensive attachment loss that can result in as much as 9-12mm in attachment loss over a six month period of time.

Typically, necrotizing ulcerative periodontitis (NUP) is found in patients who are immuno-compromised, and is a marker of immuno-suppression. It affects about 0.5% of HIV infected people, and unlike acute necrotising ulcerative gingivitis (ANUG) which is localized only to gingival tissue, it can be able to extend to the bone and supporting tissue. Necrotizing stomatitis is a severe inflammatory condition extending past the gingiva and bone and causing bone sequestration, it is associated with very severe immune compromise.[22]

Symptoms for NUP include: painful, spontaneous bleeding gums, diminished sense of taste, and metallic taste in the mouth. Gum tissue associated with this condition typically appears very red with gingival ulceration and grayish exudate in the mouth.

Treatment for NUP involves both an acute and maintenance phase of therapy. Typically, therapy that is geared towards the acute phase of therapy involves localized debridement and irrigation as well as gingival curettage. This is followed with chlorhexidine rinses that are necessary two times daily.

Antibiotic therapy involving Metronidozole and Penicillin therapy three times daily for ten to fourteen days is the typical antibiotic regimen needed for NUP, but for cases of more severe immuno-compromise, this can be changed to Amoxicillin-Clavunate (Augmentin) 875mg, two times daily for ten to fourteen days.

Maintenance phase of therapy occurs following active treatment for NUP and involves reducing infection and inflammation by debridement of infected tissue, in combination with irrigation with.12% of Chlorhexidine gluconate.

Chapter 11: Non-Surgical Periodontal Therapy

In treating periodontitis, the first line of treatment is aimed at reducing inflammation by removing plaque and its bi-products. This therapy is called non- surgical periodontal therapy.[8] It is comprised of scaling and root-planing, use of chemo-therapeutic agents such as oral rinses and use of local delivery of antibiotics as well as materials impregnated with antibacterial substances that are delivered to targeted sites in the mouth.

The use of systemic antibiotics can also be combined with non-surgical therapy to help healing and reduce chances of infection in immune suppressed patients such as uncontrolled diabetics.

Non-surgical therapy can be used to reduce inflammation and probing depth around teeth that have inflammation. Scaling and root planing involves the use of curettes and scalers, combined with ultrasonic instruments to remove diseased inflamed tissue and cementum, bacterial plaque and tartar around teeth.

During non-surgical therapy, scaling and root planing can be followed with a chemotherapeutic agent such as chlorhexidine to irrigate pockets around teeth with the goal of detoxifying and removing residual plaque film that can still stick to roots of teeth and gum tissue.

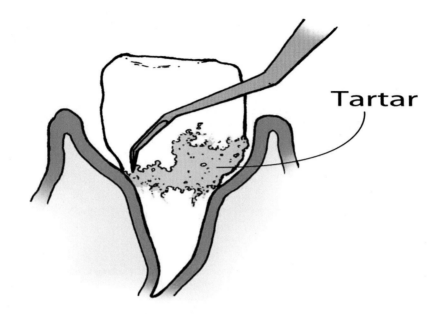

Scaling and Root Planing

Fig.19

Antibiotics can also be locally delivered to sites such as periodontal pockets and roots of teeth where they can act as an adjunct to scaling and root planing in reducing probing depth around teeth. Typically, this reduction is particularly effective especially for sites that are having probing depths up to 5mm and more. For deeper probing depths, surgical intervention in the form of flap or osseous surgery and guided tissue regeneration is usually needed.

Systemic antibiotics use in people with immunosuppression such as uncontrolled diabetics who are prone to infection can reduce inflammation and reduce their risk of infection well as aid their healing following scaling and root planing.

More recently, utilizing dental laser therapy, diseased tissue lining can be removed utilizing a dental laser, adjusted to settings to prevent damage to soft tissue, helping regenerate lost periodontal tissue and reducing probing depth.

Chapter 12: Surgical Periodontal Therapy

Following scaling and root planing the next phase of treatment is periodontal surgery for patients with persisting probing depths of five millimeters and above. Surgical therapy is also indicated when bone defects exist due to loss of bone and connective tissue surrounding teeth. Surgical periodontal therapy can be utilized to regenerate some of these defects and restore periodontal tissues to a healthier condition.

Lasers can also be used for surgical therapy and can be utilized to regenerate periodontal defects. An FDA approved procedure known as laser assisted new attachment procedure (LANAP) can utilize an FDA approved ND:YAG laser to kill bacterial pathogens reducing their numbers, and also regenerate lost periodontal attachment.[17,18]

Flap surgery involves periodontal therapy that is utilized to remove bacterial plaque and tartar under gums. It usually results in reduction of pocket depth around a tooth. Probing depth reduction and access for debridement are the end points of this procedure, and it is often enough to prevent further breakdown of periodontal condition when horizontal bone loss alone exists, and probing depth is 5mm and above.

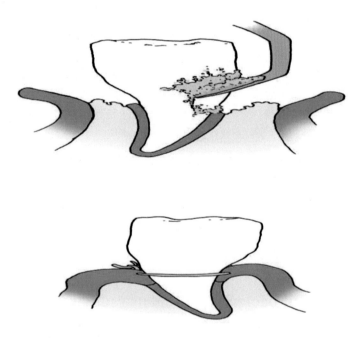

Fig.20 and Fig.21: Flap surgery

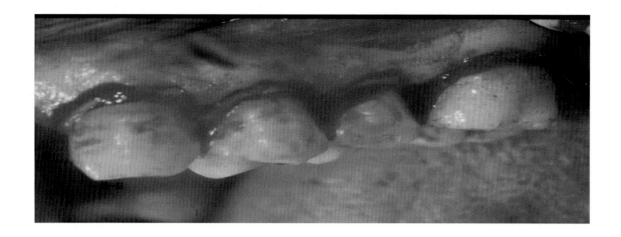

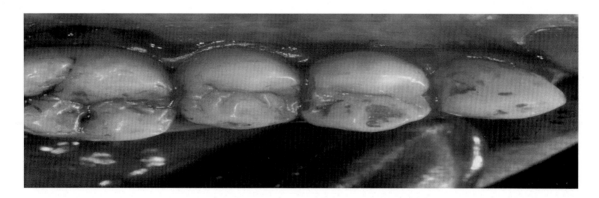

Fig.21a-c: Gingival Flap procedure showing facial and palatal incision and facial flap.

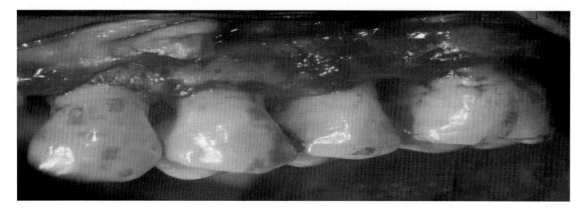

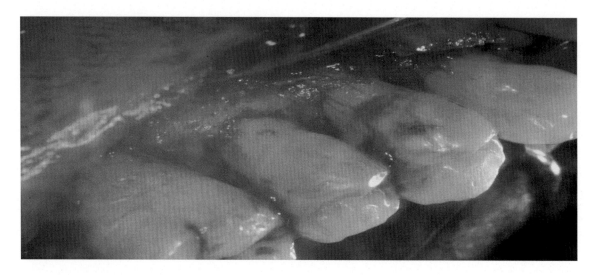

Fig.21d: Palatal flap

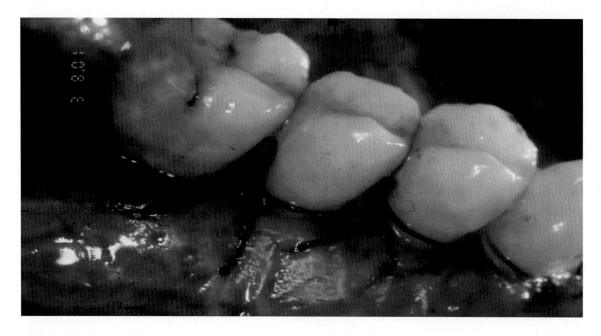

Fig.21e: Palatal sutures

Osseous surgery is a periodontal surgical procedure utilized to smooth irregularities that exist in bone around periodontally involved teeth. It is performed as part of surgical therapy where there are thick areas of bone present, or shallow crater type bone defects exist, as well as to smooth irregularities that exist in the bone as a result of bone loss. Osseous surgery also is utilized in order to reduce periodontal pockets around teeth.

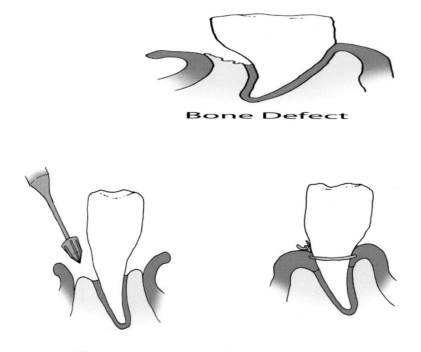

Bone Defect

Fig.22a-c: Osseous surgery procedure in which a high speed hand piece is used to adjust bone defects resulting in positive architecture that aids in probing depth reduction.

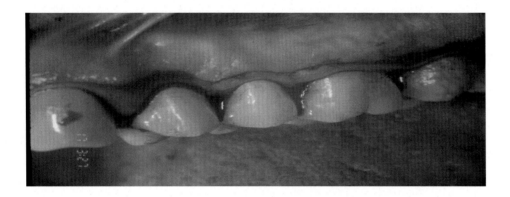

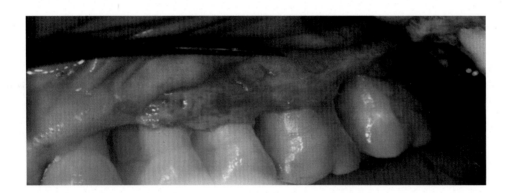

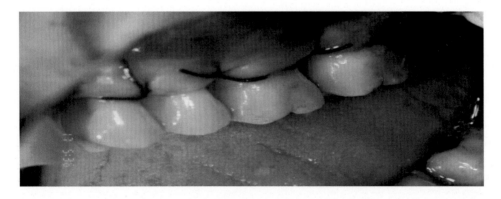

Fig.23a-c: Facial aspect of maxillary gums showing osseous surgery to smooth bone ledge and bone defects

Guided tissue regeneration surgery involves the use of bone grafts and bone substitutes as well as collagen membranes in order to regenerate bone and connective tissue attachment. During the regeneration process, lost bone, connective tissue and cementum are regenerated, improving the prognosis and stability of teeth over time. When vertical bone loss occurs around the roots of teeth, or where bone loss occurs in furcation areas of multi-rooted teeth, guided tissue regeneration surgery can be utilized to correct these defects in bone, restoring bone support around teeth.

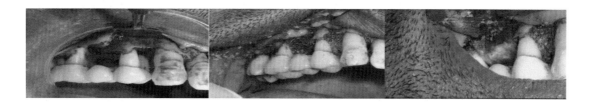

Fig.24a, Fig.24b and Fig.24c: Showing guided tissue regeneration procedure to regenerate bone for interproximal crater-like defects around teeth#3 and #5.

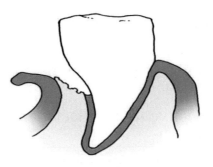

Bone Defect

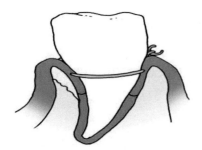

Bone Graft

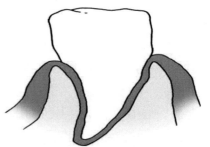

Bone Regeneration

Fig.25a-c: Showing bone grafting procedure around a lower anterior tooth

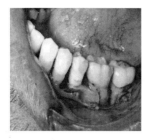

Fig.26a: Bone defect

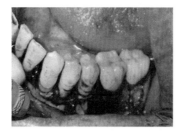

Fig.26b: Bone graft and membrane for guided tissue regeneration

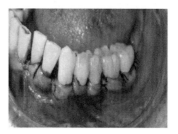

Fig.26c: Flap sutured

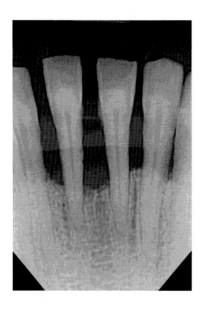

Fig.27: Before bone graft

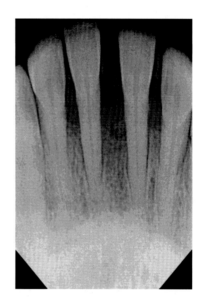

Fig.28: One year after bone graft procedure

Figures 27 and 28 show before and after pictures of bone grafting procedure done in mandibular anterior teeth. Following the bone grafting procedure, there is an increase in the bone around the teeth meaning that their prognosis has become improved as a result of increased bone support around the teeth.

Chapter 13: Periodontal plastic surgery procedures/ soft tissue augmentation surgery:

Defects in gingival tissue affecting a tooth can be able to result due to gingival recession, gingival enlargement, as well as defects in the jaws following extractions. Other defects may include Stillman's clefts which are small fissures that extend apically from the gingival margin of a tooth, that occurs typically in teeth that are in occlusal trauma. It often has the appearance of recession in those sites.

Recession defects can be caused by ectopic frenal attachments, and iatrogenic causes that can include excessive force during tooth brushing, orthodontic therapy, and oral habits, as well as deficiencies in attached tissue. Soft tissue grafting procedures utilizing donor tissue from a site that has abundant gingival tissue to augment a site with deficient gingival tissue can be performed.

The goal of soft tissue augmentation therapy is to regain attached tissue and cover recessed roots.

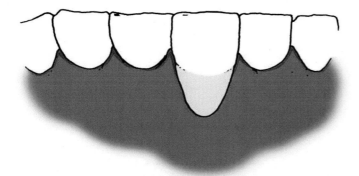

Fig.29: Gingival recession

A new classification was proposed by the 2017 World Workshop for gingival recession. The goal was to classify recession defects with regard to interdental attachment loss.[23]

1) Recession Type 1(RT1): Gingival recession with no attachment loss in the interproximal area. The interproximal CEJ is not detectable on mesial or distal aspects.[23]

2) Recession Type 2 (RT2): Gingival recession with interproximal attachment loss. The amount of interproximal tissue loss is less than or equal to buccal attachment loss.[23]

3) Recession Type 3(RT3): Gingival recession that is associated with interproximal bone loss where the amount of interproximal attachment loss is higher that the buccal attachment loss.[23]

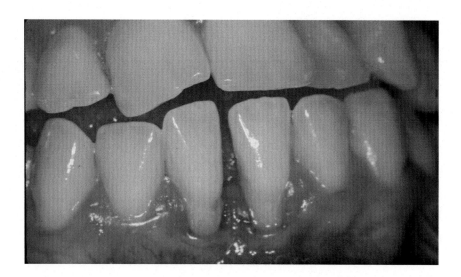

Fig. 30: Gingival recession caused by ectopic frenum attachment

Based on the desired end result of periodontal therapy, a number of periodontal plastic surgery procedures are available, and a surgical procedure that best matches the desired outcome is utilized.

The **Free gingival graft** procedure involves utilizing gingival tissue graft, from an area of the mouth where there is surplus tissue such as the palate, to another area of the mouth where it deficient. An advantage of the procedure is that there is ample tissue for the grafting procedure because there is an abundance of gingival attached tissue in donor sites like the palate.

The disadvantage of the free gingival graft procedure is that there is often a poor color match between the grafted site and adjacent tissue therefore it might not be the best procedure for esthetic areas of the mouth such as the anterior maxilla. Because it relies only on blood supply from the recipient bed only, it is also not the best technique to utilize to achieve root coverage, and is usually utilized if the goal of the procedure is increase attached tissue.

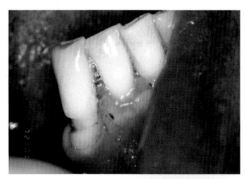
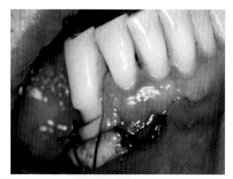
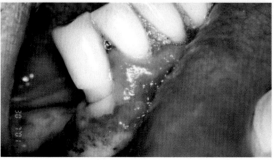

Figure 31a-c: Free gingival graft procedure

Pedicle grafts such as coronally positioned flap, lateral sliding flap and semi-lunar flaps utilize gingival tissue adjacent to the recessed site as a graft to augment the deficient tissue. They usually result in a good color match, and have good results for root coverage due to having two sources of blood supply to nourish the graft; from the recipient site as well as from the blood supply contained in the graft.

The disadvantage is that when multiple recession sites exist in a specific area, or when adjacent teeth do not have enough tissue to graft the recessed site, root coverage might not be feasible using these techniques.

As a result, the **Sub-epithelial connective tissue graft** technique utilizing sub-epithelial connective tissue in combination with a pedicle provides ample tissue by utilizing donor tissue from the palate.[9] By providing dual blood supply to the graft, the sub-epithelial connective tissue procedure is able to result in good results for root coverage, while at the same time resulting in increased gingival augmentation also as a result of the ample donor tissue.

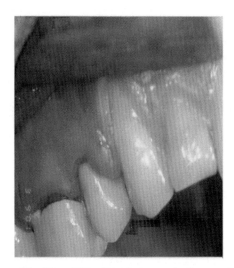 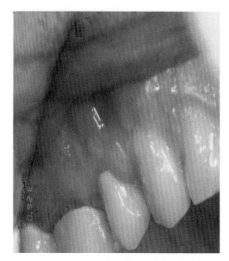

Fig. 32 and Fig. 33 : Before and after results of Sub-epithelial connective tissue graft

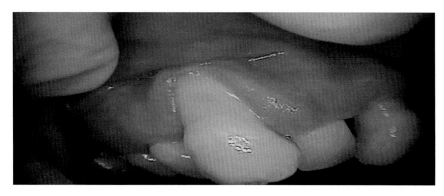

Fig. 34 and Fig. 35: Before and after results using Sub-epithelial connective tissue graft

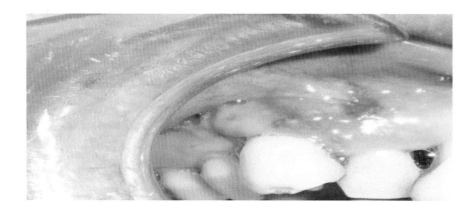

Currently, **acellular dermal graft (alloderm)** can also be utilized involving collagen tissue purchased from a donor bank that is utilized in the same way as the sub-epithelial connective tissue graft, but with the advantage of not needing surgery to harvest donor tissue. It therefore offers the advantage of requiring one surgical site instead of two, and has comparable results for root coverage with the sub-epithelial and pedicle grafting techniques. It is particularly suited for sites with multiple recession defects because there is not a limit on the amount of donor tissue that is available to utilize without removing donor tissue from the palate.[6]

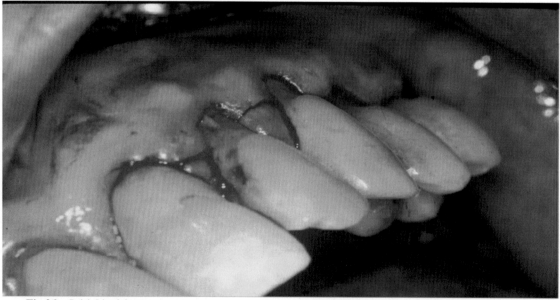

Fig.36a: Initial incisions

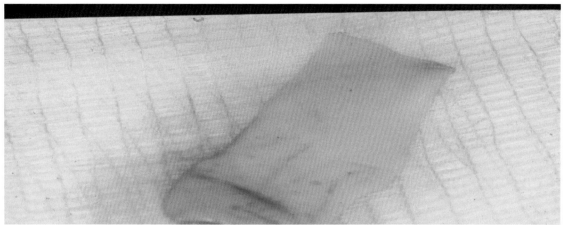

Fig.36b: Hydrated acellular dermal graft

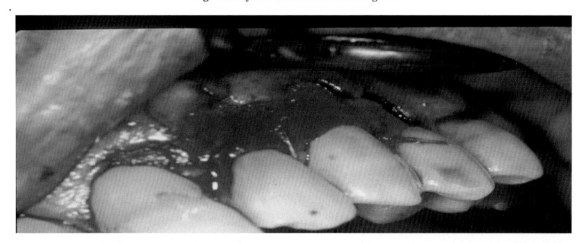

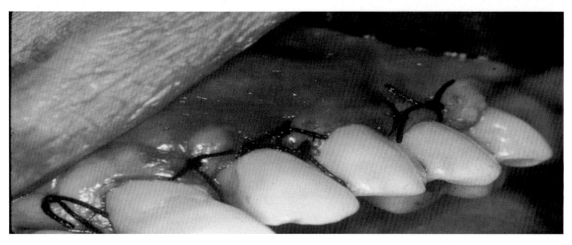

Fig.36c and Fig.36d: Sutured dermal graft and flap

Chapter 14: Dental Implant therapy

During periodontal therapy, teeth with advanced periodontal involvement may be lost. Planning their replacement is essential for people losing a tooth or multiple teeth to be able to still maintain esthetics and function. When planning to extract or replace teeth, surgical procedures that preserve the bone in extraction sockets to allow for the placement of dental implants are also important.

Augmenting the bone in an extraction socket following extraction can be performed utilizing a bone graft and membrane barrier in other to enhance bone growth in the extraction socket, and aid bone healing following extractions.

When they are defects in edentulous sites that require implants, bone grafting to rebuild bone prior to implant placement occurs through a process called guided bone regeneration. During guided bone regeneration using particulate bone grafts, bone is placed in combination with a collagen or non collagen membrane in order to regain bone for edentulous areas of the jaw that have defects in bone prior to placement of dental implants.

This allows for placement of dental implants to replace the missing teeth in sites that have optimum amount of bone for implant placement. Block bone grafts are also utilized when extensive bone loss exists in order to rebuild bone width and height prior to placing an implant.

When ridge augmentation procedures have been completed, the edentulous site is typically allowed to heal for about three to six months before dental implants are placed in the site. Dental implants are titanium screws that are gently threaded into bone and allowed to integrate with bone, in order to support functional restorations.

During the implant procedure, drills are used to prepare the sites according to the dimension of dental implant to be placed. Surgical guides aid placement of dental implants in an optimal position in bone that will allow the implant restoration to be in best position in the mouth for an esthetic result.

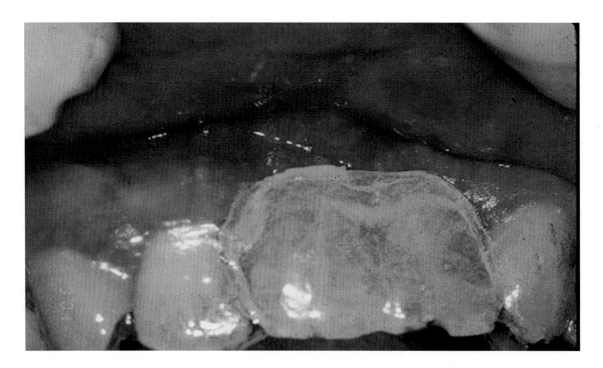

Fig. 37: Surgical guide

During implant placement, the implant is gradually threaded into bone using a very light amount of pressure, it is then allowed to mechanically anchor into bone. The implant site is sutured, and three to six months later, following a process called osteo-integration that allows bone to adhere to the implant, forming a chemical and functional bond, it is restored, replacing the previously missing tooth or teeth in the mouth.

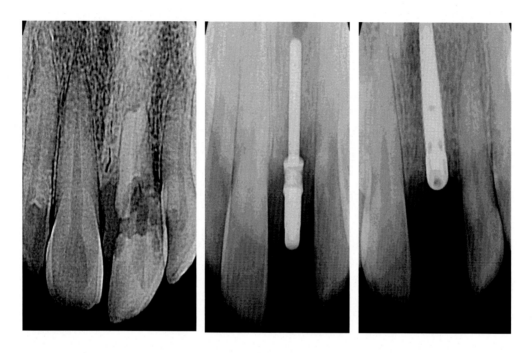

Fig. 38a-c: X-rays of dental implant placement for maxillary central incisor.

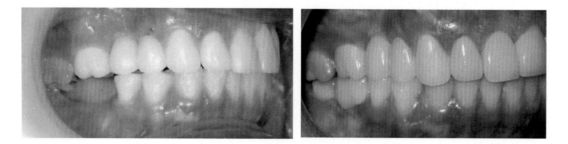

Fig.39 and Fig.40: Before and after results of posterior dental implant restorations.

Dental implant placement can occur utilizing either a single stage or two staged protocol. A single staged protocol means that immediately after the dental implant is placed, it is restored, or a healing abutment is placed to allow healing without requiring a second surgery and it is restored shortly after. A delayed or two staged approach to dental implant placement means that the dental implant is placed and restored after a period of time that can range from six weeks to six months depending method of implant restoration.

In classifying implant diseases and conditions, the 2017 World workshop indicated four categories including: peri-implant health, peri-implant mucositis, peri-implantitis and peri-implant soft and hard tissue deficiencies.[20] Peri-implant health was defined by an absence of visual signs of inflammation, and bleeding on probing. It can exist around implants with normal or reduced bone support.[20] Peri-implant mucositis is characterized by bleeding on probing and clinical signs of inflammation, it is associated with plaque, and can be reversed when plaque eliminating measures are implemented.

Peri-implantitis is caused by plaque that extends to the soft tissue and bone around implants. It can lead to loss of bone around implants, it is usually associated with poor oral hygiene around dental implants and a history of severe periodontitis.[20] If peri-implantitis is left untreated it can lead to progression and continued loss of bone and soft tissue support around dental implants.

In treating periimplantitis the goal is to control infection through debridement and use of antibiotics, in addition to also detoxify implant surfaces and regenerate alveolar bone.[25] For early peri-implantitis use of antibiotics and debridement with plastic scalers and rubber cups is usually recommended. For moderate to severe periimplantitis, implant surface decontamination using antiseptics solutions like chlorhexidine, use of air abrasion and lasers are recommended. Surgical therapy to regenerate bone is also recommended using bone grafts and membranes in combination with antibiotics such as Metronidazole and Amoxicillin.[25]

Chapter 15: Periodontal Maintenance:

Following active non-surgical and surgical therapy, another phase of therapy follows which is just as important. This phase involves maintenance of the condition of the gums in order to prevent further damage to a person's periodontal condition.

Periodontal maintenance schedule is performed typically every three months. During the visit, periodontal exams as well as x-rays are utilized to assess a patient's periodontal condition.

Changes in gum tissue can be noted, generalized scaling and prophy are typically completed at this visit, unless there is a need for additional periodontal intervention. The goal of this phase of therapy is to monitor and identify at risk sites, in order to prevent further breakdown of periodontal health.

During periodontal maintenance, occlusion is also checked so that areas that have excessive or improper contacts can be identified and treated prior to damage to the supporting structures around teeth. Traumatic occlusal forces can be able to result in damage to bone especially when inflammation is present, it is therefore important to address the inflammation when it is present. Sequential or full mouth occlusal adjustment might be necessary when heavy occlusal contacts exist, and if extensive teeth mobility is present, intra-coronal or extra-coronal splinting. Extraction of mobile teeth might be required due to excessive mobility.

Periodontal maintenance appointments also allow assessment of a patient's oral hygiene, so that habits such as excessive and aggressive brushing as well as areas that might exhibit sensitivity can be identified and corrected, and proper oral hygiene measures implemented if plaque control is lax.

Overhanging margins and other local factors that can illicit periodontal damage should also be identified and corrected during this preventive maintenance phase, prior to being able to cause further periodontal damage.

Chapter 15: Conclusion

Periodontics is the field of dentistry that deals with diseases that affect the gums and supporting tissue. A number of other conditions affect the periodontium, in 2017, the classifications of periodontal disease and conditions were reclassified under the major headings of health and gingival diseases and conditions, periodontitis, and other conditions affecting the periodontium. In defining health and gingival disease, the concept of "incipient gingivitis" which is involves localized mild inflammation that is readily returned to health following therapy was introduced. It was classified as "clinical health" which refers to tissue with complete absence of or very low levels of clinical indications of inflammation.[26] The reason behind the new definition was to have a classification of the earliest stages of gingivitis where gingival health starts to progress to gingivitis.

Other changes from the 1999 classification involved the concept of staging and grading which allows categorizing of periodontitis in terms of not only severity and extent but also on rate of disease as well as risk of progression.

Despite major efforts to diagnose and treat periodontitis, it still continues to be the number one cause of tooth loss in the United States. It also remains prevalent in general population especially for adults that are thirty years and above.

Addressing the cause of periodontal disease, by reducing bacterial plaque and its bi-products as well as reducing inflammation, has been a major goal of periodontal therapy.

This goal has become even more crucial especially with recent research indicating the detrimental effect inflammation of periodontal tissues can have on the health of other parts of the body.

By controlling inflammation in the mouth, the immune response of the body becomes enhanced resulting in an improvement in the ability to fight infection in other aspects of the body. Hence, as a result of the discovery of these systemic links with periodontal disease, recommendations were made for dentists treating diabetic patients and patients with cardiovascular disease as well as guidelines regarding screening patients with familial history of either condition.

Physicians encountering patients with both conditions or familial history of the conditions are now required to assess their periodontal condition and to refer them if periodontitis exists.[7,15] These and other developments highlight just how important reducing inflammation is to the health of the mouth and body as a whole.

A number of other factors can affect and modulate periodontitis, these factors were reviewed earlier in the book, and consist of host related versus local factors that affect the mouth. Of the host related factors, smoking appears to confer the greatest risk of periodontitis, and results in a much higher rate of tooth loss and periodontal destruction for smokers compared to non-smokers. [16]

Local factors such as overhanging or over bulked restorations which impede access for oral hygiene, as well as anatomic factors such as Stillman's clefts and cemental tears, can affect a person's periodontal condition. [10]

Occlusal factors such as traumatic occlusal contacts can adversely impact the periodontal apparatus and primary or secondary occlusal trauma can result form it. The goal is to address the cause of the traumatic occlusal contact and reduce the adverse effect on the periodontium.[24]

Peri-implant health and diseases were also reviewed by the 2017 workshop, and four categories including peri-implant health, peri-implant mucositis, periimplantitis and peri-implant soft tissue and bone deficiencies were also reviewed and just as for periodontitis, the goal is to reduce bacterial plaque around dental implants.

Systemic antibiotic therapy is playing an increased role in periodontal therapy and treating peri-implant disease, especially for treating the more aggressive forms of periodontitis that involve virulent strains of bacteria, which cannot be eliminated by scaling and root planning or surgery alone and for treating periimplantitis. By adding systemic antibiotic therapy to periodontal therapy, the ability of a host to fight bacterial infection caused by these strains is enhanced.[8]

More recently, DNA tests have been produced that help identify bacterial strains so that they can be targeted by antibiotics geared towards the specific bacterial strain.

Localized antibiotics can now also be utilized in conjunction with scaling and root planning to reduce inflammation and probing depth around teeth and implants. Significant reduction in bleeding and probing depth parameters were noted compared to scaling and root planing alone.

For surgical therapy, a number of innovations have also been made such as enhancing bone grafting materials by adding peptide proteins to aid bone regeneration as well as utilizing enamel matrix proteins to further enhance bone growth during guided tissue regeneration.

For gingival grafts, a-cellular dermal grafts provide the added advantage of reduced post-operative discomfort as a result of requiring one surgical site instead of two. They eliminate the need for use of donor tissue from sites intra-orally with comparable surgical results as connective tissue grafts.

All of these measures have contributed to surgical and non - surgical therapy and are advances that have helped to facilitate the treatment of periodontal disease and restoring the health of periodontal tissues.

References:

1) Albander JM et al. Destructive periodontal disease in adults 30 years of age and older in the United States 1988-1994. J of Periodontology 1999. Jan;70(1):pp 13-29.

2) Armitage GC. Development of a Classification system for periodontal diseases and conditions. Annals of periodontology 1999;4: pp1-6.

3) Armitage GC. Periodontal Diagnoses and Classification of periodontal diseases. Periodontology 2000;34(2004):pp:9-21.

4) Bollen CML and Quirynen. Microbial response to mechanical treatment in combination with adjunctive therapy. A review of Literature. J.of Periodontology 1996, vol 67(11) : pp 1143-58.

5) Brenan RM and Genco RJ et al. Bacterial Species in sub gingival plaque and oral bone loss in post-menopausal women. J. of Periodontology 2007; 78:pp 1051-1061.

6) Drisko Connie. Trends in Surgical and Non surgical Periodontal treatment. JADA. June 2000 vol.131.No 1supplement 1:pp31S-38S.

7) Friedevald V, Kornman K, Beck J et al. Editors' Consensus Report on Cardiovascular disease. J. of Periodontology 2009; 80: pp 1021-1032.

8) Greenstein G. Non surgical Therapy in 2000: A Literature Review. JADA Nov 1, 2000 vol 131(11):pp1580-1592.

9) Langer et al. Sub-epithelial connective tissue graft technique for root coverage. J of Periodontology 1985. vol 56:pp717-720.

10) Leknes KN. Influence of anatomic and iatrogenic root characteristics on bacterial colonization and periodontal destruction: A review. J. of Periodontology 1997. June, 68 (6): pp507-566.

11) Loeshe et al. Periodontal disease as a specific chronic infection, diagnosis and treatment. J. of Clinical Microbiology Rev.2001;14(4)pp727-752.

12) Lovegrove JM. Dental plaque revisited: Bacteria associated with periodontal disease. JNZ Soc. Periodontology 2004; 87:pp 7-21.

13) Prichard JF. Management of Periodontal abscess. Oral Surgery, Oral Medicine, Oral pathology, Volume 6, Issue 4, April 1953. pp 474-482.

14) Reinhardt R et al. Influence of Estrogen and osteopenia/osteoporosis on clinical periodontitis in post-menopausal women. J. of Periodontology 1999; 70 (8):pp 823-828.

15) Southerland J et al. Diabetes and periodontal infection:- making the connection. Clinical Diabetes 2005;23(4): pp 171-178.

16) Tomar SL and Asma S. Smoking- attributable periodontitis in the United States, findings from NHANES III. J. of Periodontology 2000; 71 (5):pp743-751.

17) McCawley T et al. Lanap Immediate effect in vivo on human chronic periodontitis microbiota. American Dental Research 33rd Annual meeting2014, Abstract 428.

18) Nevins et al. Human clinical and histologic evaluation of laser assisted new attachment procedure. International Journal of Restorative Dentistry 2012; 32:pp 497-507.

19) Murakami S et al. 2017 World Workshop. Dental plaque-induced gingival conditions. Journal of Periodontology.2018;89(Suppl.1):S17-S27.

20) Caton JG et al. 2017 World Workshop. A new classification scheme for periodontal and peri-implant diseases and conditions- Introduction and key changes from the 1999 Classification. Journal of Periodontology 2018.(89(Suppl.1):S1-S8.

21) Todescan S et al. Necrotizing Ulcerative Gingivitis. Journal of Canadian Dental Association 2013;79: d46.

22) Papapanou PN et al. Periodontal consensus report of workshop2 of the 2017 World Workshop on Classification of Periodontal and Peri-implant diseases and Conditions. Journal of Clin. Periodontology.2018;45(Suppl 20):S162-S170.

23) Jepson S et al. Periodontal manifestations of Systemic Diseases and

Developmental and Acquired conditions. Consensus report of the Workshop 3 of the 2017 World Workshop on classification of periodontal and peri-implant diseases and conditions. J of Clin. Periodontology 2018.;45(Suppl.20):S219-S229.

24) Fan J et al. Occlusal trauma and Excessive occlusal forces: Narrative review, case definitions and diagnostic considerations. J of Clin. Periodontology 2018; 45(Suppl.20):S199-S206.

25) Prathachandran J et al. Management of Peri-implantitis 2012. Dental Research Journal.2012 Sept-Oct;9(5):516-521.

26) Lang NP et al. 2017 World Workshop. Periodontal Health. J.of Clin. Periodontology.2018;45(Suppl.20):S9- S16.

Printed in the United States
By Bookmasters

Periodontitis is the number one cause of tooth loss in the United States for adults thirty years and older. Periodontal disease affects over seventy-five to eighty percent of adults, and more recently has been found to have major implications for systemic health especially for patients with diabetes and high blood pressure. In 2017 the American Academy of Periodontology (AAP) and the European Federation of Periodontology (EFP) collaborated to create a new classification for periodontal disease and peri-implant diseases. The goal of this revised edition is to review this classification and contrast it to the 1999 classification as well as evaluate its impact on periodontal diagnosis, prognosis and therapy.

Understanding Periodontitis not only reviews the categories of periodontitis, but also provides a detailed informative resource on diagnosing, categorizing and treating periodontitis. By utilizing illustrations as well as actual pictures of various procedures, it works well also as an interactive informative hand book that dentists, hygienists, as well as dental patients alike will benefit from to better understand periodontal disease.

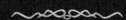

Dr. Obiechina completed her training in periodontics and implant dentistry from Columbia University in 2001. She received her doctorate in dental medicine degree from University of Pittsburgh in 1998. She is the recipient of the Melvin Morris award for clinical excellence from Columbia University in 2001, as well as the Northeast Regional Board Student award for excellence in periodontics.

She has worked extensively within the field of periodontics with two goals in mind: To offer periodontal and implant therapy that is non-invasive and state of the art, as well as to educate patients and people in general about periodontal disease and it detrimental effect on dental and overall health.

She has been practicing all scopes of periodontics and implant dentistry in the east and west coast for the last 17 years and has active licenses in New York, DC, New Jersey and California.

authorHOUSE®

ISBN 978-1-4634-4611-6

56500

9 781463 446116

Run Benny Run!

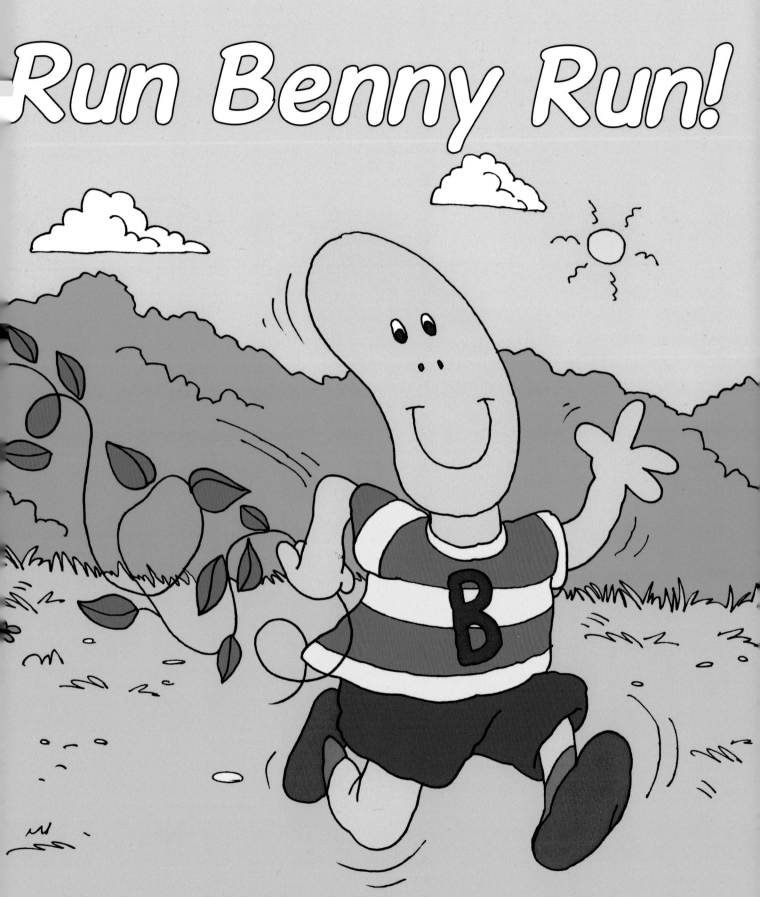

written by Kathy Bingham Powell